Swee
Note

Ideals Children's Books • Nashville, Tennessee

Sweet Surprises

Each message in this delightful collection was designed to be given to a sweetheart or spouse. Fifty-two tear-out notes come in three varieties:

Special Days • Awards and Coupons • Thoughts and Promises

Because laughter and fun are important to a relationship, *Sweet Surprises* will help you express your feelings—often with a humorous touch! So tear out a note and then . . .

- Tuck it in a briefcase or purse for an at-work surprise.
- Slip it under a pillow for an early morning treat.
- Hide it in the refrigerator with a favorite snack.
- Or simply pass it along with a kiss!

Copyright © 1995 by Hambleton-Hill Publishing, Inc.
All rights reserved. Printed and bound in the U.S.A.
Published by Ideals Children's Books • Nashville, Tennessee 37218
An imprint of Hambleton-Hill Publishing, Inc.
ISBN 1-57102-051-9

Special Days

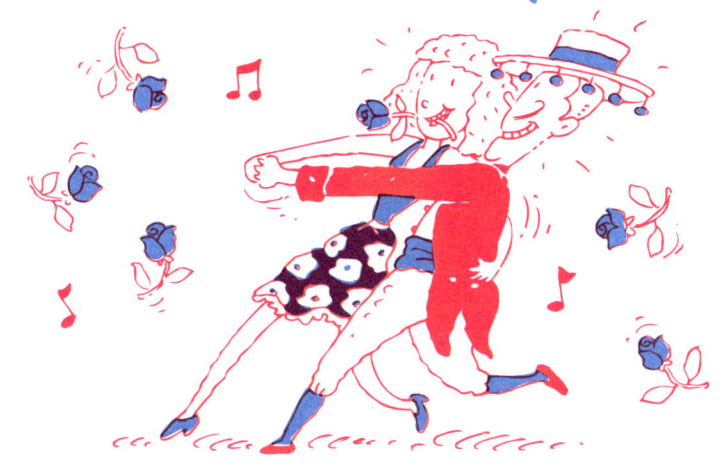

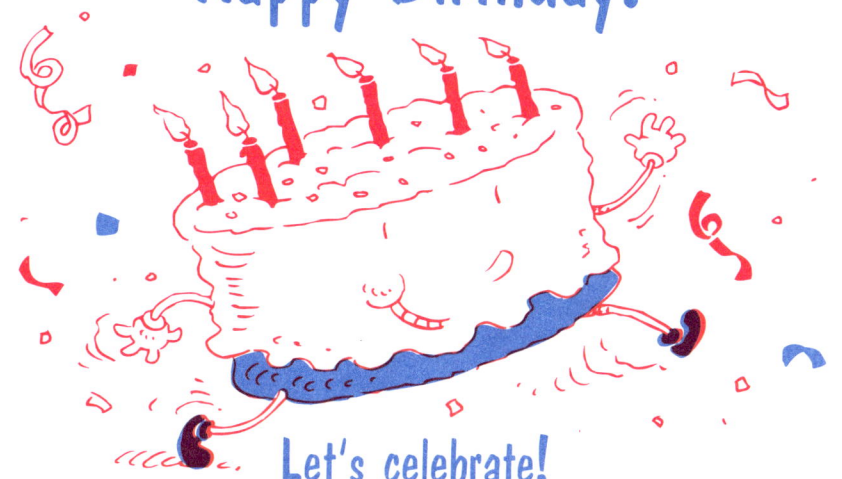

To: _____

From: _____

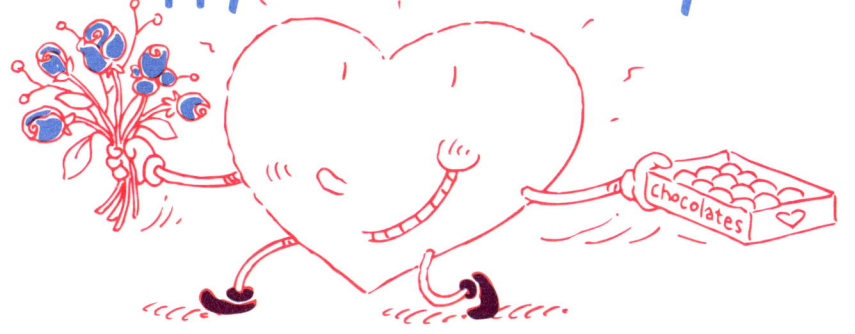

To: _____

From: _____

Awards and Coupons

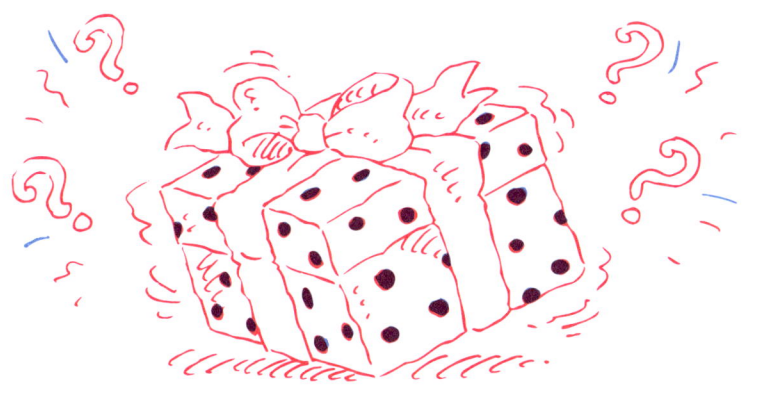

This coupon is good for one night
out on the town
with the best date around—ME!

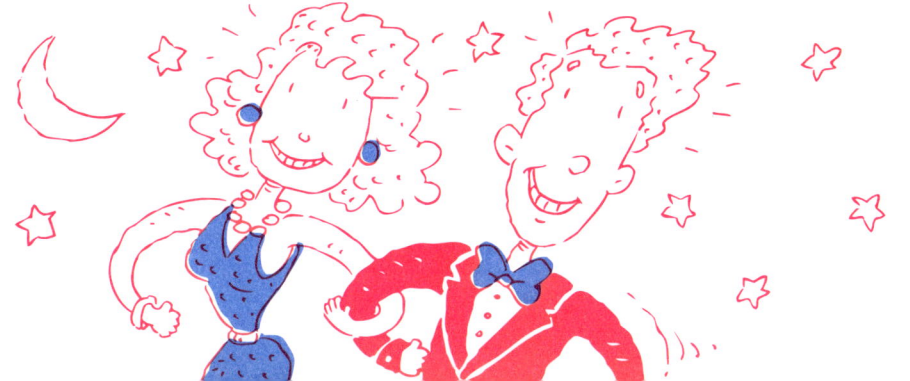

To:_____

From:_____

The bearer of this coupon is entitled to one breakfast in bed.

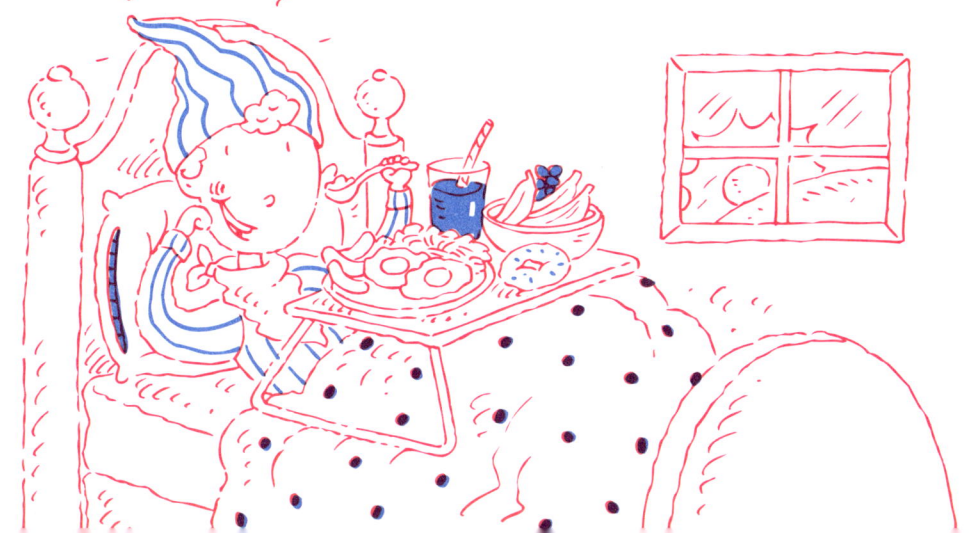

To: _____

From: _____

The bearer of this coupon is entitled to a romantic rendezvous.

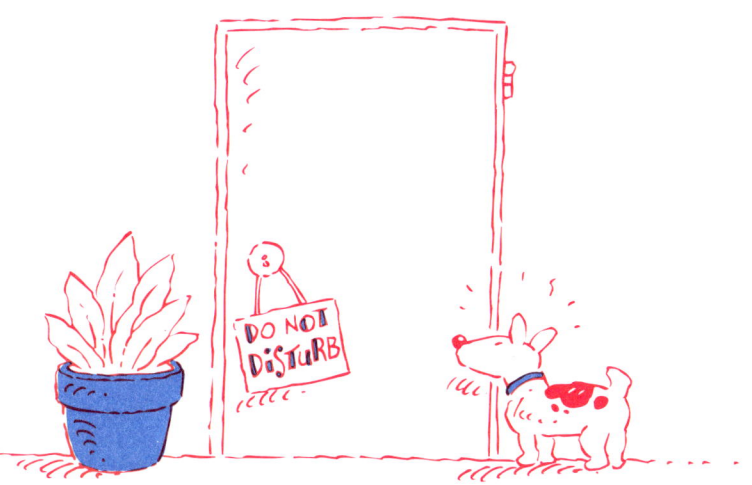

To:_____

From:_____

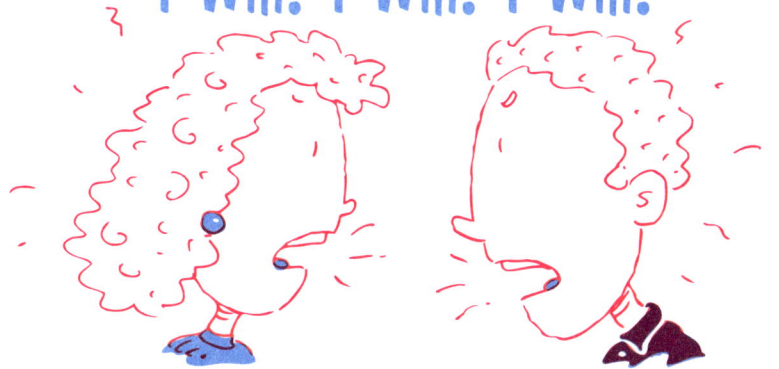

To: _____

From: _____

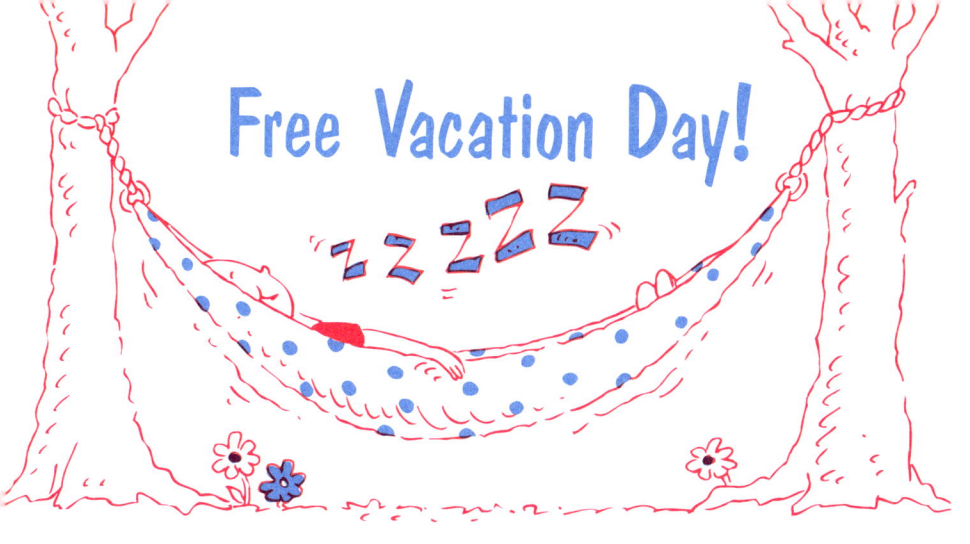

To:_____

From:_____

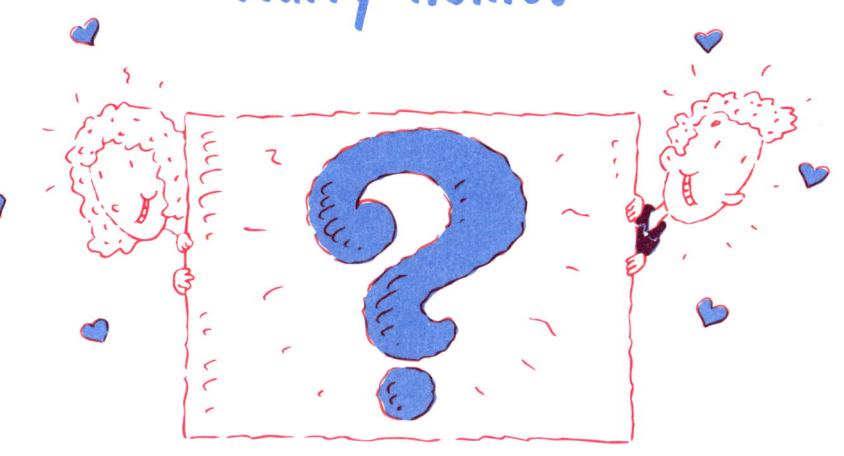

To:_____

From:_____

It's Your Day!

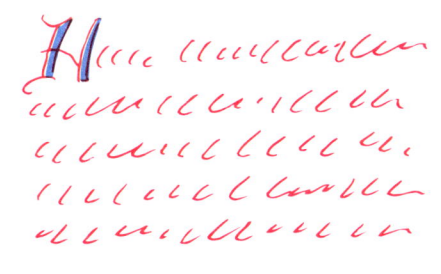

Official _____ **Day**

In celebration of this occasion, _____ is entitled to one day of complete at-home pampering and total indulgence.

To:_____

From:_____

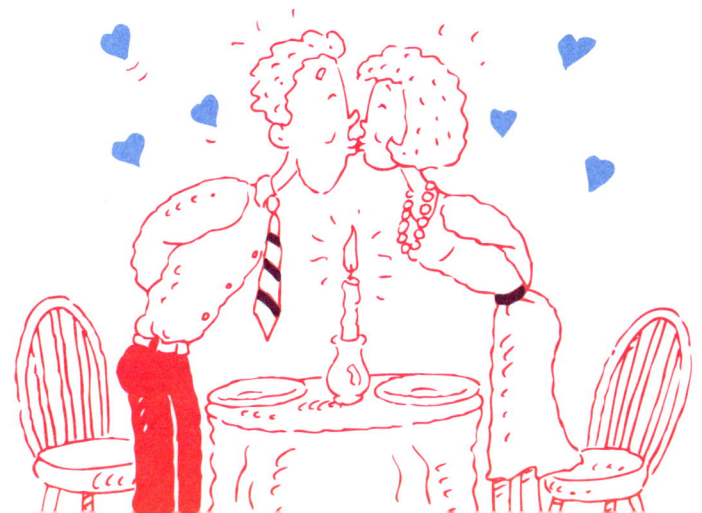

To: _____

From: _____

This coupon may be redeemed for one bubble bath—complete with candles.

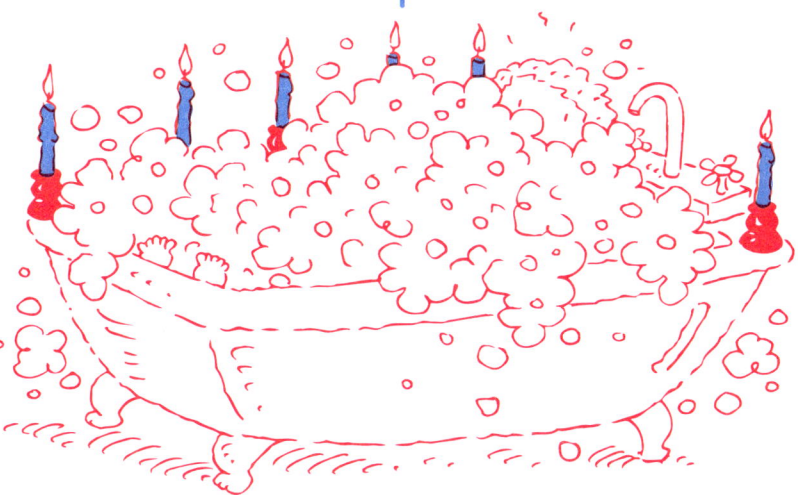

To: _____

From: _____

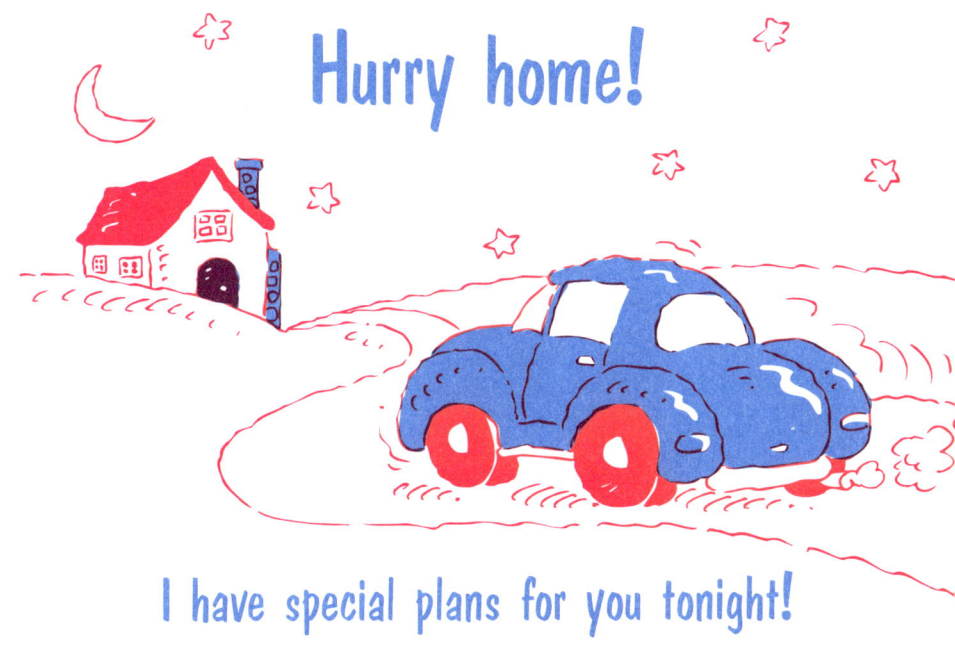

To:_____

From:_____

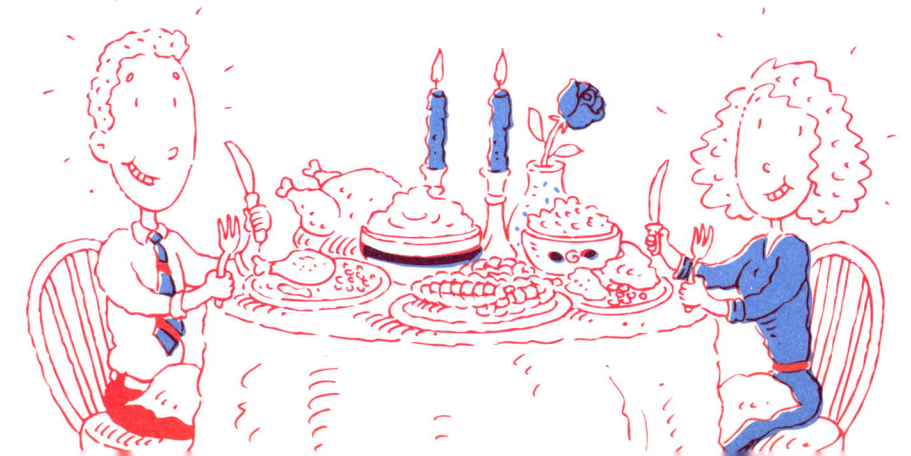

To:_____

From:_____

Today is officially declared
Get Your Way Day!

You get your way all day!

To: _____

From: _____

I've planned something special just for you.

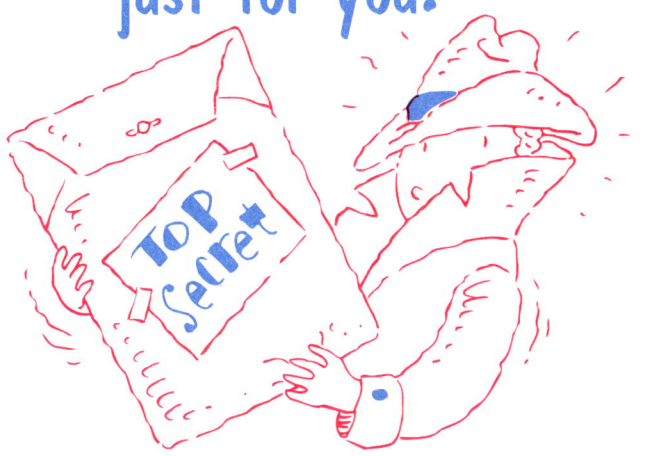

To: _____

From: _____

Turn in this coupon for a mystery surprise!

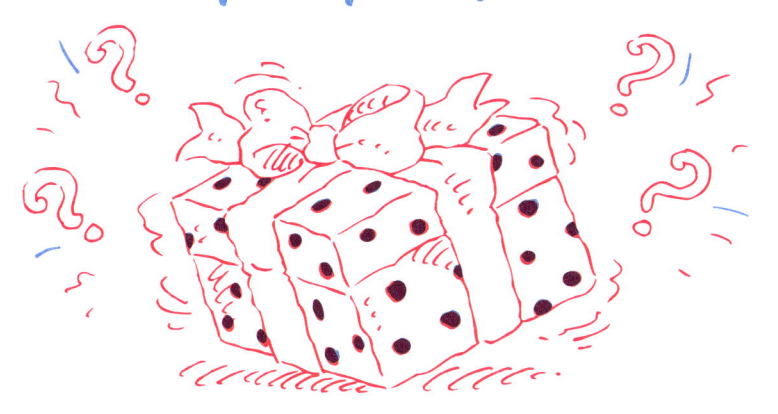

To: _____

From: _____

The bearer of this coupon is entitled to

_____

_____

_____

To: _____

From: _____

The bearer of this coupon is entitled to

_____

_____

_____

To:_____

From:_____

Thoughts and Promises

Let's Celebrate!

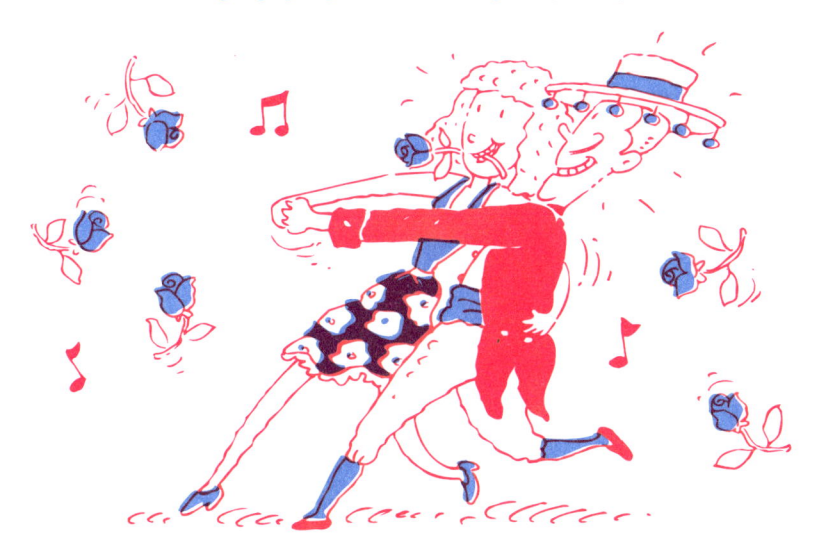

To: _____

From: _____

I'm proud of you.

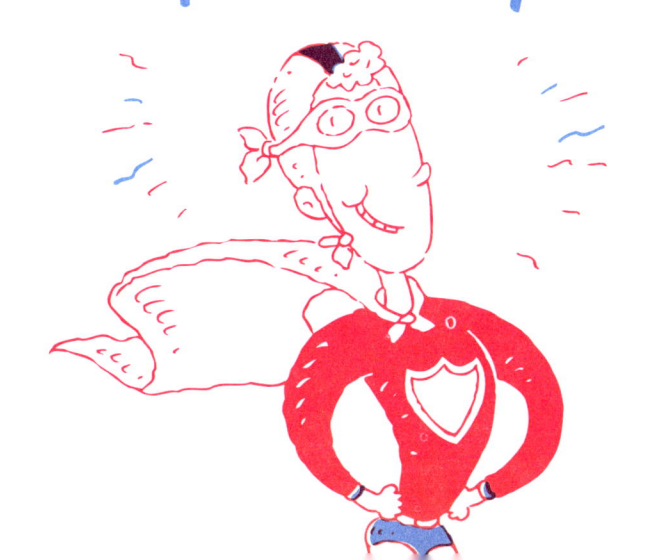

To:_____

From:_____

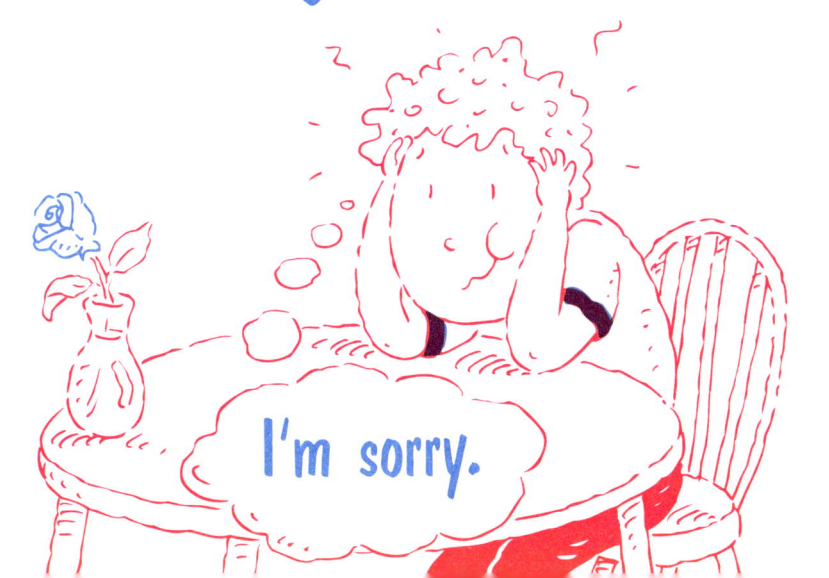

To:_____

From:_____

Just a little note to say—
Hope you have a wonderful day!

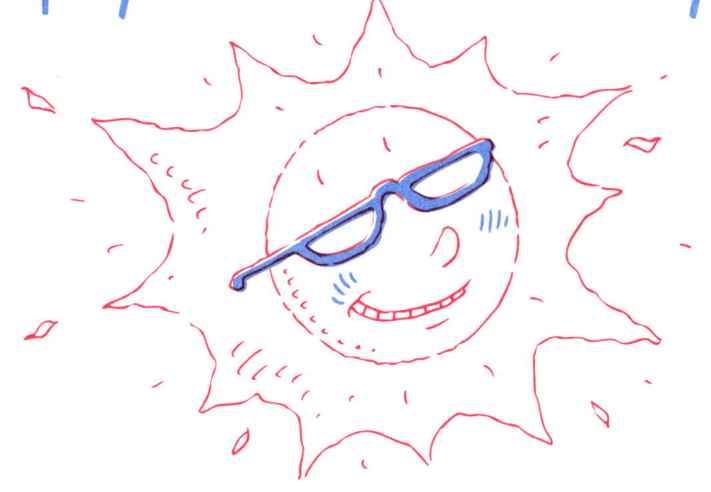

To:_____

From:_____

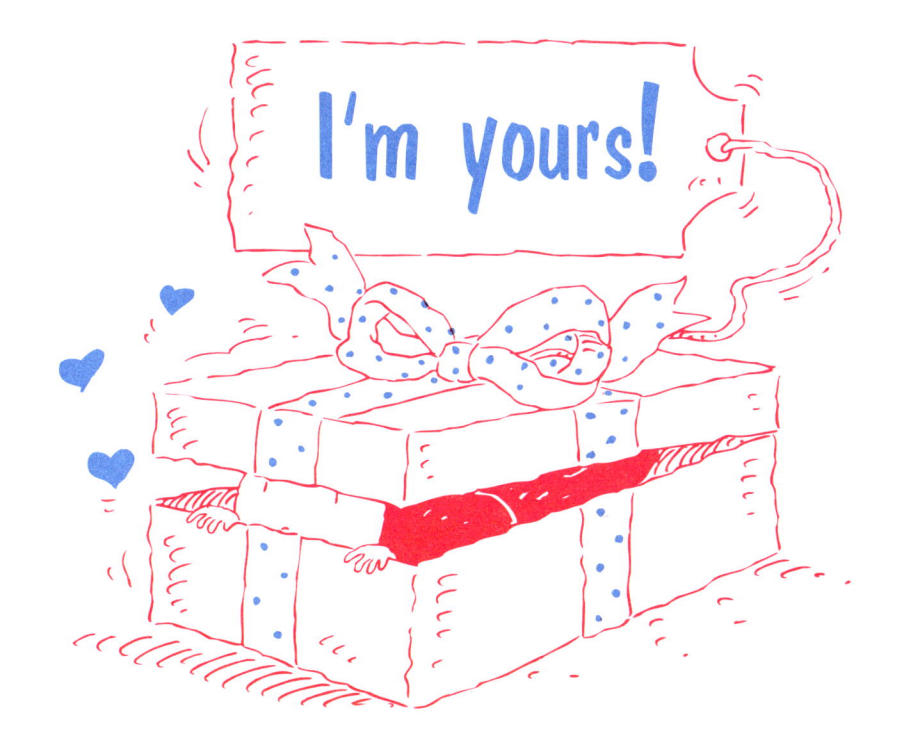

To: _____

From: _____

Happy Anniversary!

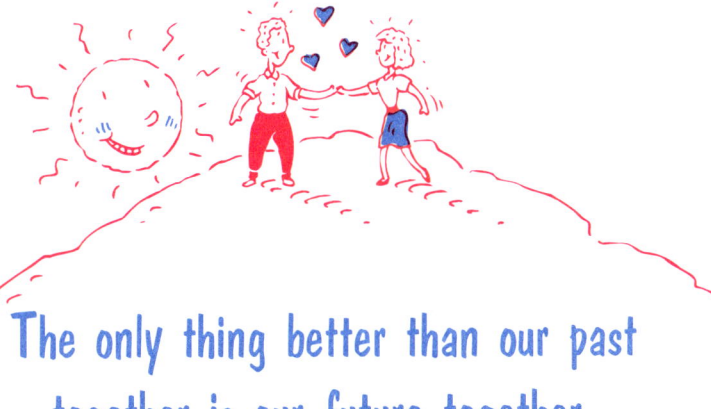

The only thing better than our past together is our future together.

To: _____

From: _____

I know you can do it!

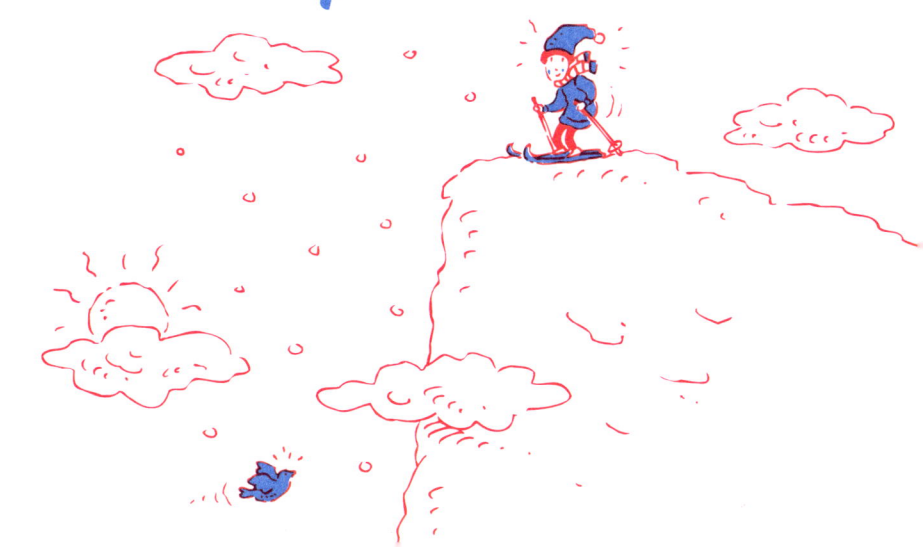

To: _____

From: _____

Good Luck!

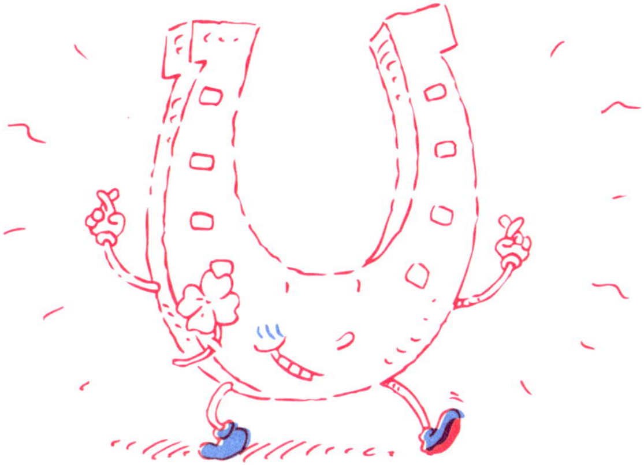

You'll do great.

To:_____

From:_____

If you want to talk, I want to listen.

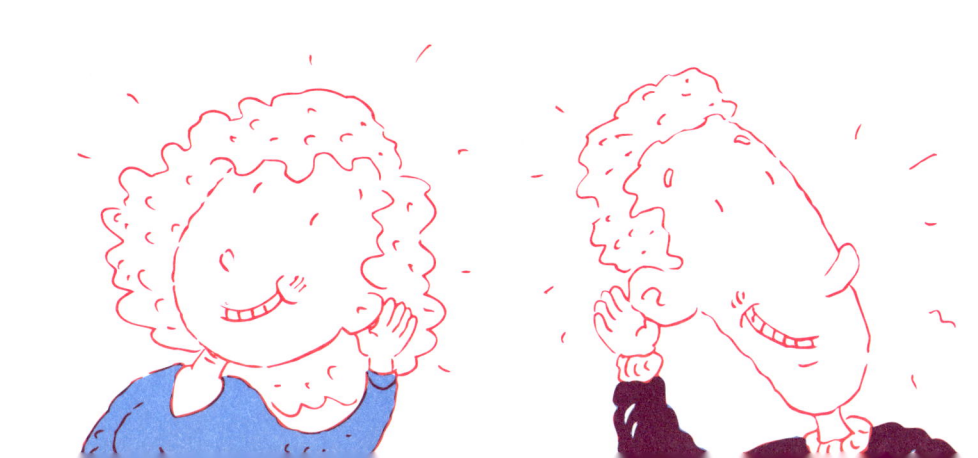

To:_____

From:_____

For all that you are,
For all that you do—
With all of my heart,
Thank you.

To:_____

From:_____

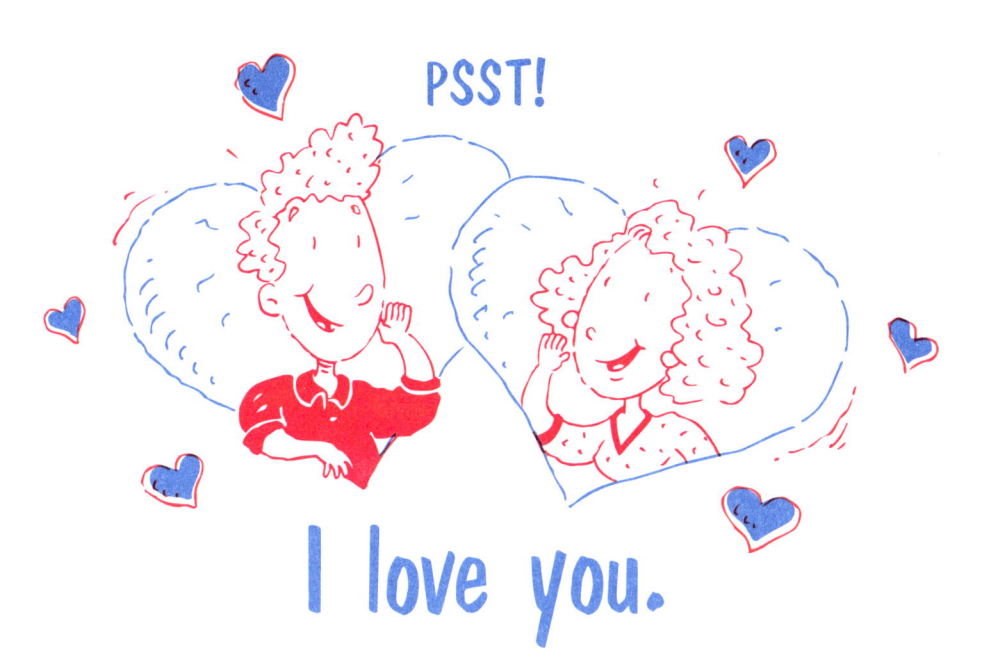

To:_____

From:_____

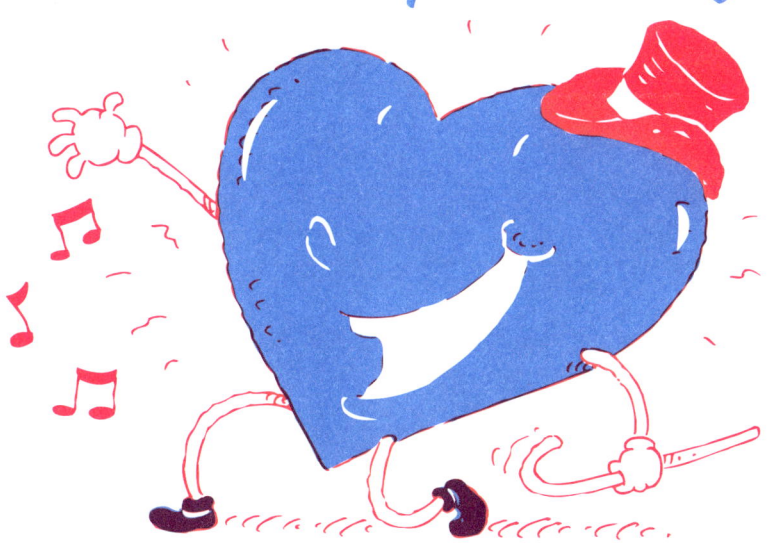

To: _____

From: _____

Sometimes even I make mistakes.

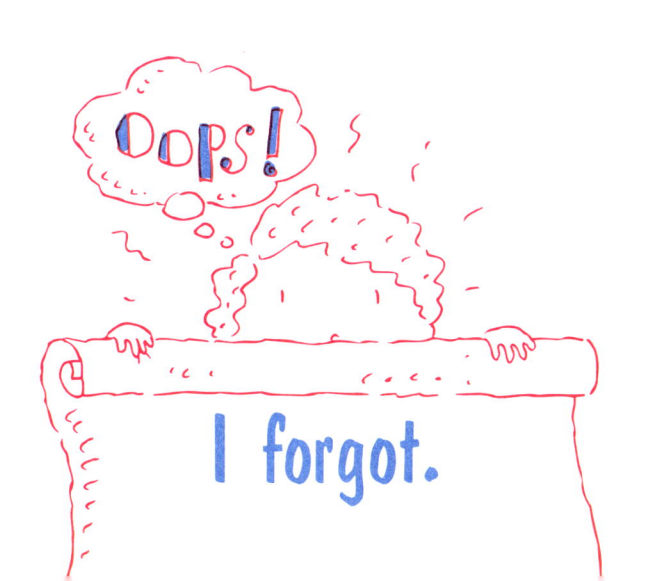

OOPS!

I forgot.

To: _____

From: _____

Cheer up!

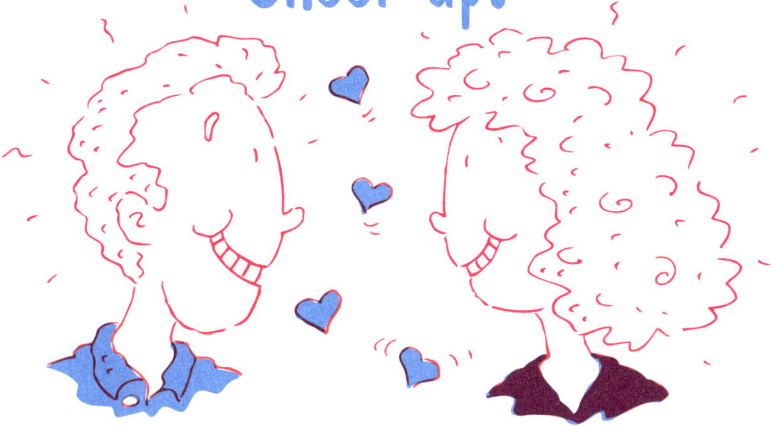

We'll do something special tonight!

To: _____

From: _____

Congratulations.

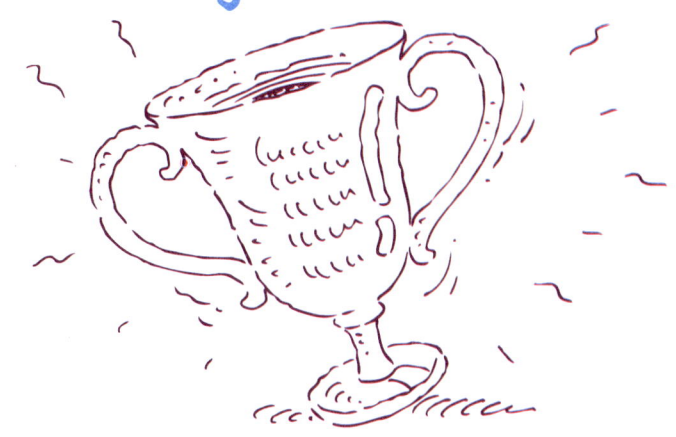

I know how hard you've worked for this.

To:_____

From:_____

And now—those magic words you've been waiting for—

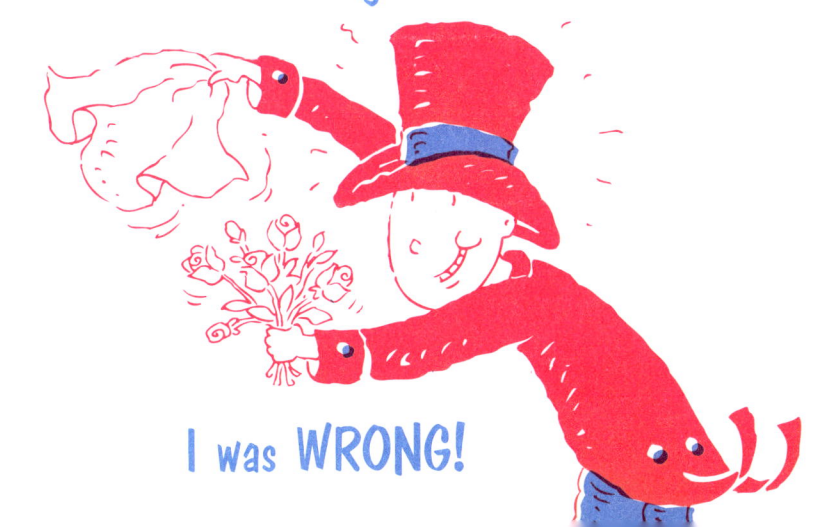

I was WRONG!

To:_____

From:_____

Hope you feel better soon!

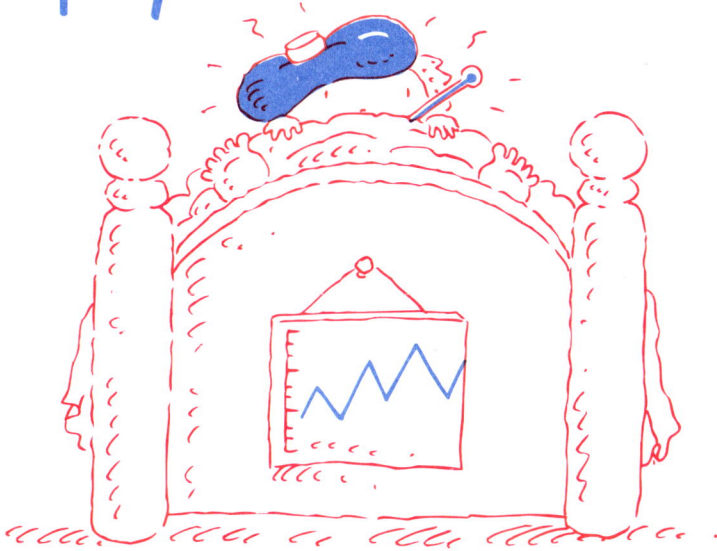

To: _____

From: _____

I was right!

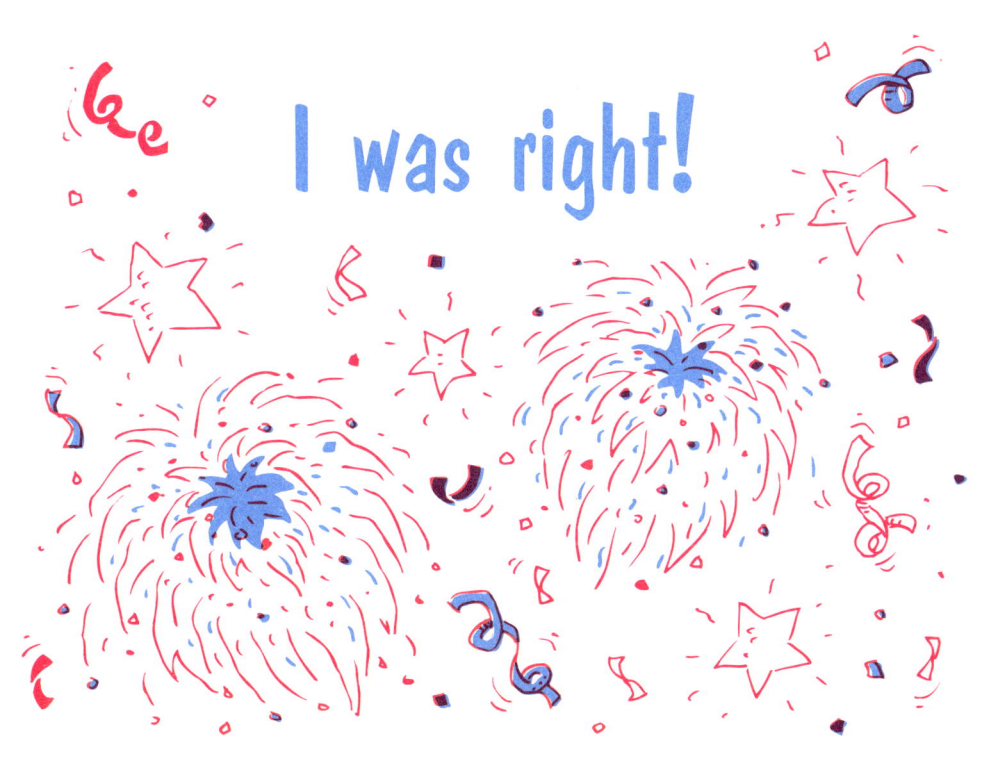

To: _____

From: _____

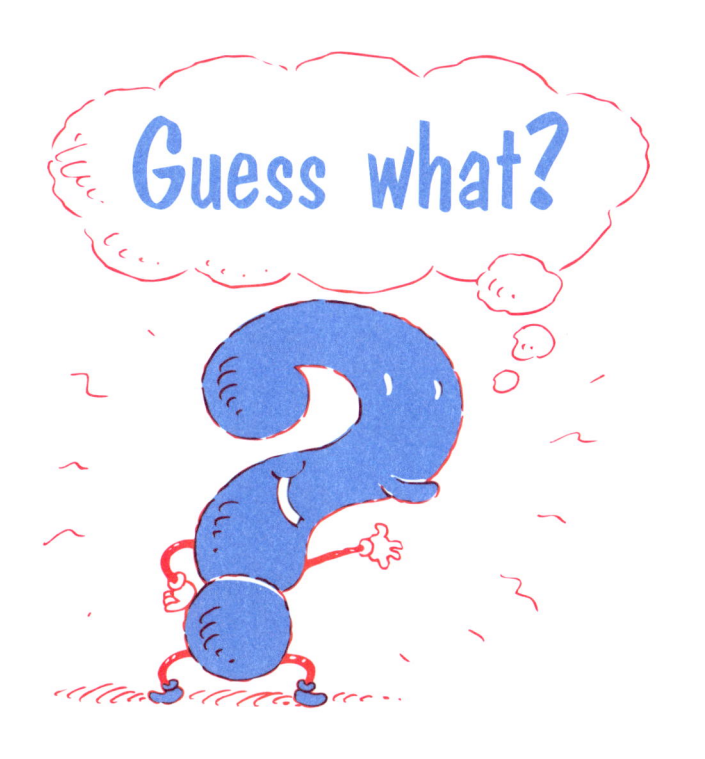

To:_____

From:_____

PSST!

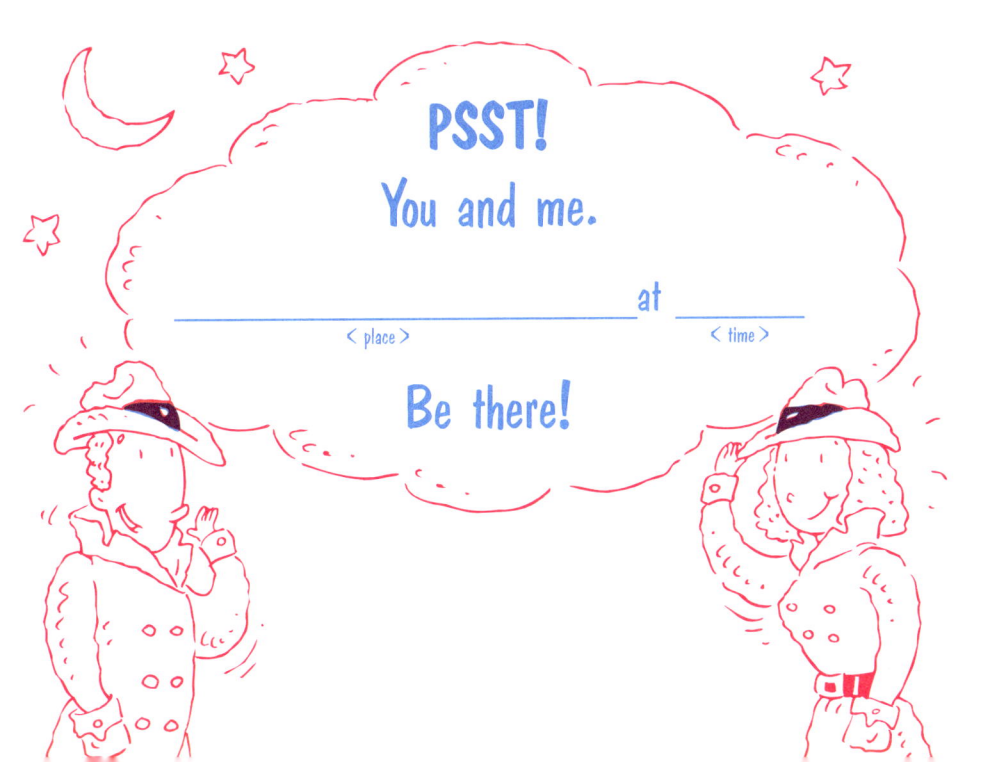

You and me.

_____ at _____
  〈 place 〉   〈 time 〉

Be there!

To: _____

From: _____

A loving thought from me to you . . .

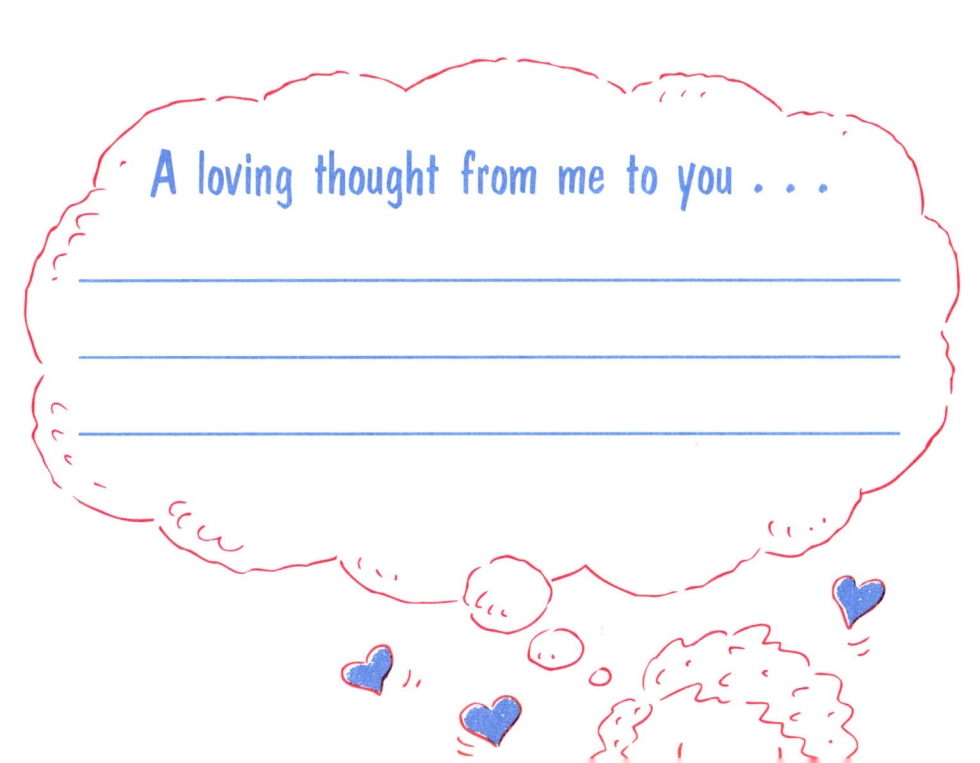

_____

_____

_____

To:_____

From:_____

A loving thought from me to you . . .

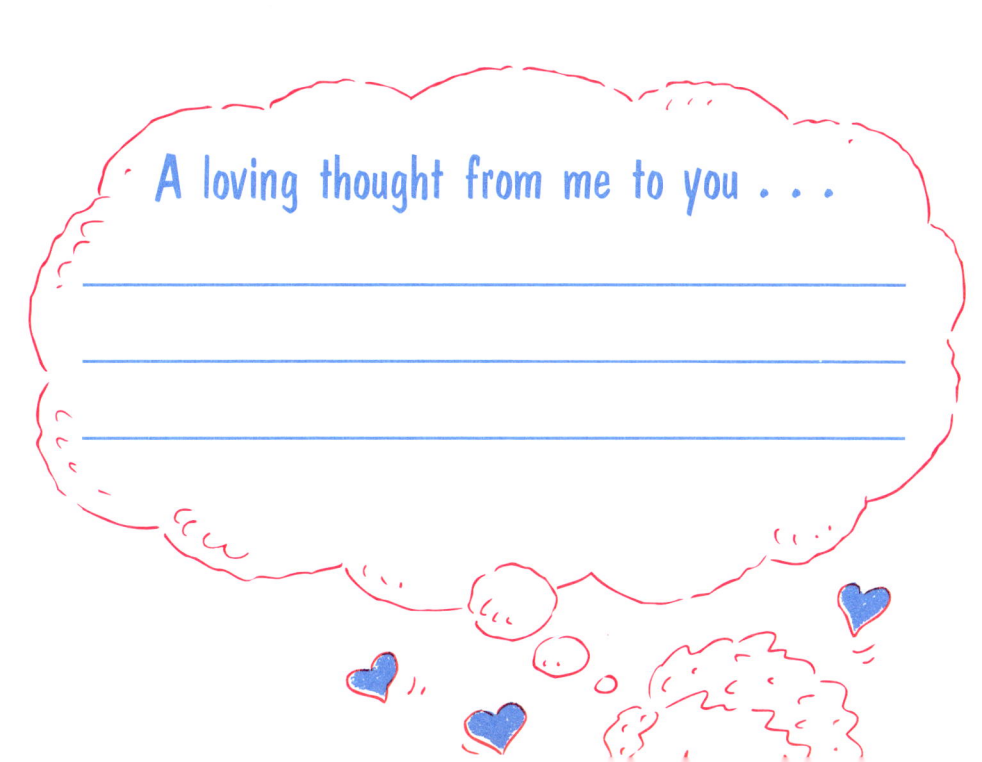

_____

_____

_____

To: _____

From: _____

A loving thought from me to you . . .

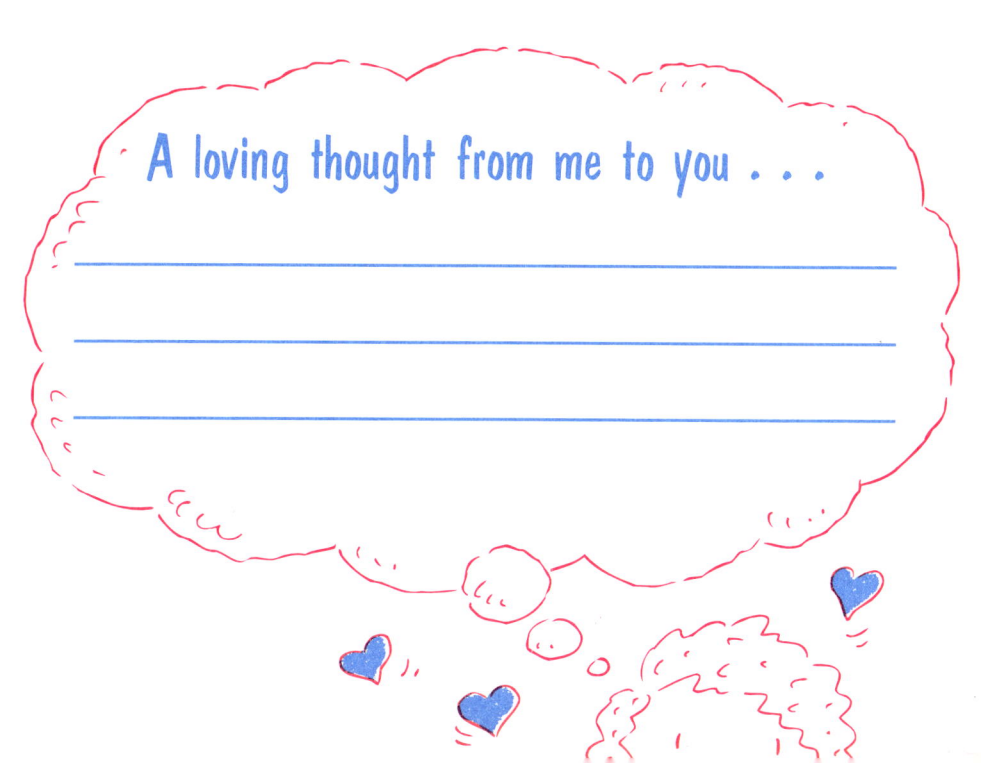

To: _____

From: _____